1. Spectrum, plant life cycles, and macular degeneration

2. Green light and its significance

3. Far red application and how it influences phytocrome Pr & Pfr

4. PPFD and photon distribution to canopy

5. Future improvements to expect from LED manufacturers

6. Cooling fans and heat syncs, pros/cons of LEDs not having fans

7. Secondary optics and transmittance test

8. Photosynthetic rates with only 450 & 660nm wavelengths

9. LED emitters 1, 3, & 5 watt

10. Ideal PPFD levels for the different amounts of CO2 and UVB

1. Is there an ideal spectrum for the entire lifespan of the plant, or is it better to have different spectrum for different phases of a plants lifecycle? Like more blue for vegetative and additional red for flowering cycle? Or is one continuous spectrum better? What are some of the pros and cons of each? What's the best way to create a comparison of grow lights?

"Gregory Goins from Kennedy Space center has done research on growing leafy vegetable plants onbaord a spacecraft. For long missions, it will be very useful for astronauts to grow their own salad type veggies such as Spinach, radish and lettuce. In his 2001 article he has used red LED with blue light supplementation and in his 2005 articile he has used red and blue LED;s with green light supplementation from Florescent light (In 2005, green LED did not exist)."

Solar System 550 California Light Works

"In neither one of these articles, or any other article I have read on grow light I have read anything about different recipes for different phases of the vegetable growth. He has used the same recipe throughout from planting to harvest. Probably the only thing that one has to be careful about is when the leaf grows it gets closer to the light source, so one has to adjust the light intensity to make sure the ppfd remains the same. There may be another philosophy which recommends changing the light recipe at different phases, but I don't know anything about it."

Using the Lighting Passport and SGAL will be the best way for grow lights to be compared. The software program allows for PPFD comparison at nanometer specific wavelengths, making the Lighting Passport an ideal spectrometer for those searching to optimize their horticulture facility and the energy it consumes.

Comparison using SGAL

While reading these research papers there was no study found where different spectra were used at different phases of the plants growth cycle. There are consistent treatments for the entire life span of the plant. Yet, one of the most sought after characteristics of a LED is spectrum adjustment capability, and this is because each species and strain has its own set of individual spectra needs. With LED spectrum adjustment capability on a fixture the number of plant species one could grow increase.

https://www.researchgate.net/publication/10938361_Improving_spinach_radish_and_lettuce_growth_under_red_LEDs_with_blue_light_supplementation?enrichId=rgreq-596baf40-8189-454b-a084-56fbfe52c637&enrichSource=Y292ZXJQYWdlOzEwOTM4MzYxO0FTOjE5ODU2NDg1MzYyMDczNkAxNDI0MzUyOTU4MzY4&el=1_x_2

The July issue of Max Yield in 2010 had an article that sparked my interest in LED technology. It explains that; "most growers know that plants are more responsive to red light in the flowering stages of growth, and blue light for vegetative phases."

One of the major advantages of LED technology is using the specific wavelength needed to influence a photosynthetic response from your plants. Lighting Science and VividGro are very interests in researching lighting recipes for different strains and varieties.

"Because LEDs can emit specific wavelengths, growers can now optimize lights for plant growth. By mixing various LED chips, a complex light spectrum can be created for different growth conditions."

"Aside from chlorophyll and photo pigments that drive photosynthesis, plants contain a variety of photoreceptors that sense and utilize light. These include crytochromes, phytochromes, and phototrophins. Each react to different wavelengths and the ratio of their active and inactive forms cause different reactions in plants. At various stages of plant development different light conditions are required for different lengths in time."

<u>Max Yield July 2010 by Brian Chiang and Josh Pucket</u>

"When plants grow leaves, they optimize the leaves for the light they are currently receiving. <u>Whenever light intensity or spectrum changes, the existing leaves aren't optimized for the new conditions, and the plant undergoes shock.</u> Leaves grown under the new lighting conditions will be optimized for it, but until new leaves grow the plant isn't able to best use the new light it's getting. By using the same spectrum for vegetative and flowering cycles, we eliminate this shock, and have noticed a decrease in flower time (1-3 days) and an increased yield when the plant was grown for its entire life under one spectrum."

"Plants grown under a red-heavy spectra for flowering tend to get leggy with weak stems. In nature, the upper canopies of plants block most of the blue light, but the far-red light penetrates to lower leaves and other plants. Plants that want full sun have evolved to encourage rapid stem growth when exposed to a low blue-to-red light ratio-- this makes them increase inter nodal spacing to grow tall and try to "stretch through" whatever is shading them out. By including the right ratio of blue light throughout flowering, inter nodal spacing is shorter, stems stay stronger, are less prone to breaking, and the plant expends less energy growing stems, and more energy producing flowers or fruits.

F1 tomato & red flame peppers under a Solar System 550

"Using LEDs, we can fine-tune, down to the nanometer, the light we are providing the plant. Our Phytogenesis Spectrum provides the correct ratios of blue to red, and far red light (even UV) to encourage the plant to stay compact while growing and flowering vigorously."

PhytoMAX-2 800 in a test setup 4x4 with 6 plants

"The result is higher quality and quantity of plant growth at the same time, without sacrificing efficiency or falling into the old "blue for veg, red for flower" way of thinking."

https://www.blackdogled.com/faq-about-black-dog-led-lights#veg-and-flower-spectrum

Macular Degeneration- Is the harmful effects to the retina. When we thing of LED lighting and the fact that a LED focusing its illuminance on 450nm and 660nm, we realize it can be much different than being in the sun for example. So, naturally our eyes have to make an adjustment. As the cones respond to different wavelengths of light the BLUE is particular interesting.

www.Alliedscientificpro.com

"The retina of the human eye does not handle blue light well. Doctor Sliney states that blue light sends an extremely intense signal to the muscles of the eye telling them to shut down. It can cause severe headaches and nausea. Intense blue light is also capable of causing permanent photochemical damage to the eye. The LED lights, whether white, blue, infrared, or ultraviolet, are very bright and can be intense enough to injure human eyes."

"It's worth mentioning for grower safety that working under poorly engineered LEDs that are red-blue spectrum only quickly lead to eye strain and headaches and should be avoided. Also, the flicker in some cheap units is an outright health concern as it can induce seizures in some individuals." Fortunately the SGM software app has a built in flicker test which can be used to make sure no fixtures are damaged and flickering which will improve the environment safety for employees working under the lighting systems.

[Zondits Interview with Peter Rumsey, Executive Vive President of Sales and Business Development of LightingScience/VividGro](#)

These thoughts on spectrum bring us to our next topic which is green light and its purpose in a facility. Still a controversial topic today in 2017 because plant physiologists have different methods and philosophies on what are optimum conditions for certain genetic varieties.

F1 tomato flowers under a V2 from Lighting Science

2. Any thoughts on green light will be very useful. Is it beneficial to incorporate this portion of the spectrum in an indoor horticulture fixture? Reb/blue seems to have pros and cons, and the white light LEDs have a different set of pros and cons. it seems green light helps penetrate the canopy, although when I think of a LED fixture; is it worth consuming electric to have the green section for indoor horticulture?

"Best is to read Gregory Goin's paper on using red, blue, and green for growth. The link is available at the end of the book. It seems that addition of green light to red and blue will have the following advantages"

"Under red and blue, the appearance of plants looks purplish grey which makes any visual assessment of any problems or defects very difficult. Addition of green light will make it possible to produce a natural white light and the makes the visual inspection much easier. However my point is that for a space mission, the astronauts may benefit from looking at the natural colors of the plants but if the plant is grown on earth, one can only operate the red and blue lights and when you need to inspect the plants turn on a set of white lights. The white lights or the green light need not be on all the time in my opinion."

"There is the issue of penetration of green light deep into the Canopy. If you look at McCree reference, you will see that although you will see that red and blue have bigger peaks, green also has a weight, So in a bushy environment, the leafs below can benefit from green light. However as far as I know, if you are growing lettuce or Spinach, there are not too many bushes and the concept of penetration deep into the Canopy does not apply.

"Figure 2 in Gregory Goin's 2005 paper (attached here) shows that when he compared several different lamp configurations in growing lettuce, the red,blue, green gave 30% more Leaf area Index and Crop growth rate as compared to Red and Blue only. However the question is if it is worth it to have green light on and pay for electricity to get this extra growth?

"As far as I have seen in most of the veggie growth facilities and show demos, most of the big horticultural light companies, only use blue and red and not green. I would say it is **better not to use it.**"

It seems balancing resources consumed with green light delivered to the canopy will be an issue that deserves proper contemplation by those building the PFAL. It interesting how there is research showing the benefit from green light like how plants are more resistant to disease for example. Yet, many LED manufacturers leave it out of the spectrum or keep green light at a very low PPF. This would suggest that the answer to our question is NO we should not burn resources to give green lght, or a lot of green light to our plants in controlled environments. Still, the real question is will green light be necessary for your canopy?

"Although YPF and the amount of absorbed light were higher in the RB treatment, the RGB treatment resulted in greater biomass production."

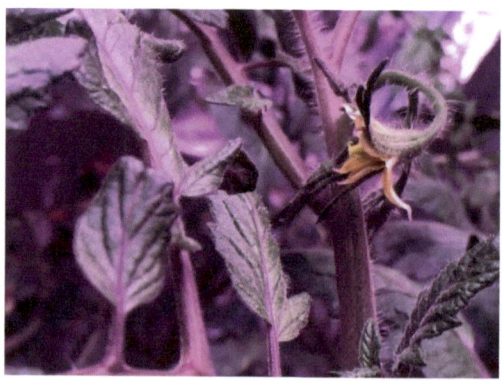

Early Floral Development under a V1

https://www.researchgate.net/publication/7963634_Green-light_Supplementation_for_Enhanced_Lettuce_Growth_under_Red-_and_Blue-light-emitting_Diodes?enrichId=rgreq-13a41f01-a70b-4445-9b30-c21e575245d9&enrichSource=Y292ZXJQYWdlOzc5NjM2MzQ7QVM6MTk4NTY0ODUzNjIwNzM4QDE0MjQzNTI5NTkwMDc%3D&el=1_x_2

H-19 Little leaf OG Cucumber trial

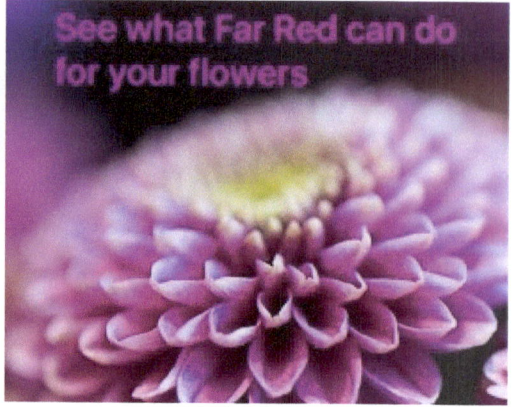

<u>F1 under a Solar System 550</u>

"Red plus blue light appeared purplish gray, and disease and disorder became difficult to diagnose. Lettuce plants with and without <u>5% green</u> from LEDs with both treatments at the same total PPF. They observed no impact on lettuce growth with all measurable characteristics such as photosynthesis rate, shoot weight, leaf area, and leaf number being the <u>same with and without green</u>"

"They also used red and blue LEDs with and without green fluorescence (GF) at <u>24% green for RGB, or 0% green for RB</u>. This experiment demonstrated that lettuce plants grown with RGB had higher fresh and dry weights and greater leaf area than those grown with RB alone"

"Light sources consisting of more than 50% green caused reductions in plant growth, whereas combinations including up to 24% green enhanced growth for some species."

http://hortsci.ashspublications.org/content/43/7/1951.ful

"The question of how much green light is absorbed and used in photosynthesis by the green leaves of land plants has therefore been solved. By considering the intra-leaf profiles of light absorption and photosynthetic capacity of chloroplast."

"The wavelengths with strong absorption, the loss of absorptance by the sieve effect is large. On the other hand, at wavelengths of week absorption such as green, the loss is marginal. The sieve effect, therefore, strongly decreases absorptance at wavelengths of strong absorption such as red and blue light.

Spectrum Lab

"The increase in absorptance due to light diffusion is significant in the spongy tissue in bifacial leaves whose abaxial surface are paler than their a diaxial surfaces. In such leaves spongy tissues have cell surfaces facing various directions and fewer chloroplasts or chlorophyll per unit mesophyll volume."

"Green leaves absorbed much green light. Typical values of absorbance at 550nm range from 50% in Lactuca sativa to 90% in evergreen broad leaved trees. The corresponding absorptance values for blue and red lights range from 80-95%."

https://oup.silverchaircdn.com/oup/backfile/Content_public/Journal/pcp/50/4/10.1093/pcp/pcp034/2/pcp034.pdf?Expires=1493256339&Signature=V5DVH6t5d7nSO5feZ~Zfv0X78Audop7MZLsVjibqCqDzMXUg9hmcPUXD9tdlUKV7TNLJhTlYDpGSVqKbyt3kj0g4uIoErfidLbVCe9xriD5OcSiUsjHvRB6uFTtRsi1Ef2fZgC51ZP2BNO~DFTE1KVdQl8teBuHre~TDvs1iFrBM3bSq9AQgmhoauJ7hI0IzoH6GoUUcLrKjYfq57stKEEJcbcboGermjadPiNO4~BMWoM8DxgcqJ-I0II32rpqYzOgt9rY2f9b2jXyfCpXPaRwv9c0HKaYnypW-YtrlVMt-7SzZMB1q3qnkkIId~9qDHDHtM9Lhh4YfUhHpqTJ-g__&Key-Pair-Id=APKAIUCZBIA4LVPAVW3Q

"While it is true that green light is mostly reflected by the chlorophyll in plant leaves (this is why they look green), this doesn't mean plants don't use any green light. Other pigments in leaves such as carotenes and xanthophylls harvest some green light and transfer it to the photosynthetic process. The small amount of green we include also serves as an aid for viewing the plants, allowing easier diagnosis of issues such as nutrient deficiencies, pest and disease problems."

https://www.blackdogled.com/faq-about-black-dog-led-lights#veg-and-flower-spectrum

Lighting Science focuses on this topic but from a different perspective. One that I was surprised to hear, yet very impressed with. When building facilities one must balance plant needs with worker needs. LEDs that grow great plants may make an uncomfortable working environment for gardeners. Since growers must work in these facilities its ideal to optimize the entire business model. Always wear number five welders sunglasses, Ok?

"One more critical advantage to Lighting Science grow LEDs is that we have also, as a result of our work with NASA, optimized our LED grow fixtures to be "highly palatable" to human vision for those who must work under and around them. Due to our optimization efforts, we not only improved the horticulture performance, but also created a spectrum that is easy and pleasant to work under and around."

Zondits Interview with Peter Rumsey, Executive Vive President of Sales and Business Development of LightingScience/VividGro

"Addition of green LED light resolves this problem for human vision"

http://hortsci.ashspublications.org/content/43/7/1951.full

Another point that should be brought up is that observation and analysis of nutrient deficiencies are much more difficult under a red blue only spectrum, some LED manufacturers like Lumigrow and California Light Works add a view mode for inspection. Since the spectrum created by lighting science is optimized for human eyes, it's also much better to make observations in the work facility. Please keep this point in mind as we move forward with these questions because after question four we will observe the spectrums and see an example.

3. Any additional thoughts or research paper links concerning "far red" 730 nanometer specifically? Should this be incorporated into a LED spectrum? It seems far red can be used to influence the length of day and allow growers to keep the lights on 14/10 instead of 12/12 using an EOD (end of day) treatment. Any thoughts on this? Previous studies? Also since far red influences the phytocrome Pr & Pfr; should a LED spectrum have far red continuously lit (all day) ? What are your thoughts on the differences if any between far red 730nm and 760nm.

http://growlightsource.com/products/the-flower-initiator-and-booster-grow-lights/

"There are two additional links from research papers at the end, one by Kubata (I think it should be 2011) and another by Strutt (2009). I have not heard anything about FR influencing the length of the day. So I am not sure about about this one. <u>However I know that FR at 730 nm influences the morphology of the plant and activity of phytochromes</u>."

"In the two papers referenced at the end they have used it as a constant supplemental light source for lettuce (specifically) and they have also used at the <u>End of the Day (EOD) treatment for seedling (For example 30 min EOD for three days). This has caused extending stems for seedlings and expanding leaf and enhancing growth rate for leafy greens</u>."

Far red LEDs can be used in maximizing photosynthesis, photomorphology, and photoperiodic control. Far Red LEDs specifically 735 nanometer in wavelength can be used in horticulture for a photoperiodic and used as supplemental photosynthetic lighting. The Far Red with a response peak of 735nm is a light quality relevant to plant growth and development. LED lighting also allows for monochromatic far red lighting.

For example supplemental far red lighting has shown expanding leaf and enhancing growth rate in leafy greens. Also in PFAL growth chambers there has been extending stem/hypocotyls of plants especially seedlings. Far red is effective at a very low intensity.

Supplemental far red light significantly increased the biomass of baby lettuce plants by 28%. This was due to the increased light interception caused by enhanced leaf elongation, and there have been similar observations by Struttle et al. (2009).

Applications of Far-Red LEDs in Plant Production under Controlled Enviroments **Chieri Kubota**

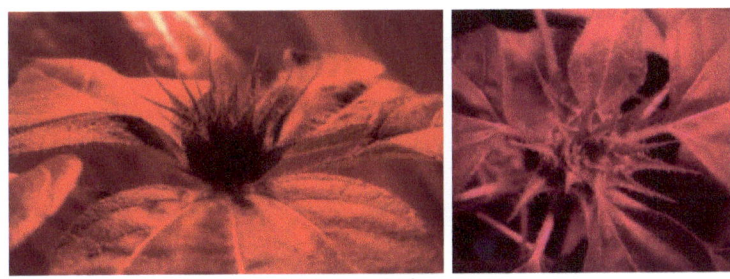

Strawberry Blond F1

"Phytochromes are a family of proteins that have two forms, red absorbing form (Pr) and the far red absorbing form (Pfr). The Pr form, which has λmax = 660nm, undergoes a conformational shift to the Pfr form when it absorbs light. The Pfr form which has λmax = 730nm, undergoes a conformational shift to Pr when it absorbs light. The Pfr form is generally considered to be the active form (Smith and Whitelam, 1990)."

"Also, be very concerned about the relative balance between the $\lambda = 660$ and $\lambda = 730$nm in the light source. The most relevant factor in photobiology is the fraction of the phytochrome present in the active Pfr form with resoect to the total phytochrome (P tot = Pfr + Pr) at photoequilibrium."

"The phytochrome state (Φ) is established by multiplying the irradiance (N) at each wavelength (λ) against the relative absorption at that λ for each form of phytochrome."

http://hortsci.ashspublications.org/content/44/2/231.full

"Far red light, is important for stimulating flowering of long day plants (Deitzer et al., 1979;Downs, 1956) as well as for promoting intermodal elongation (Morgan and Smith). The blue light photoreceptor class of cryptochromes has been found to work in conjunction with the red/FR phytochrome photoreceptor class to control factors such as circadian rhythms and de-etiolation in plants (Devin et al., 2007)"

http://hortsci.ashspublications.org/content/43/7/1951.full

"The proportion of mesocotyl tissue was significantly higher for seedlings grown with IR, whereas the proportion of coleoptiles tissues was significantly lower. An ancillary observation was that the IR LED radiation made seedlings significantly straighter and trained them to the gravity vector, and the authors proposed a gravitropism photon-sensing system with potential involvement of phytochrome (Johnson et al,. 1996). Better productivity generally is seen with additional wavelengths and broadening of the spectrum."

http://hortsci.ashspublications.org/content/43/7/1951.full

4. When we observe measurements of PPF and PPFD which is more applicable to horticulture? What is the significance of each and why is the actual photon distribution so important? Which is more applicable to HID lights, and which is more accurate in measuring the efficiency of LED horticulture fixtures? Should researchers use the same methods for testing all forms or artificial lighting for horticulture?

"I definitely prefer using ppfd to ppf. ppfd is like Irradince which is most important. A lamp can have a large ppf but if the surface to be illuminated is far away, it will receive less ppfd and the plants won't grow."

Let's look a little bit deeper into exactly what is meant by these two figures PPF and PPFD; The following reference from the scholarly articles is great, although the saying from the VP from Lighting Science in the following paragraphs was the best explanation I've heard throughout this entire research and writing process.

"PPFD (Photosynthetic Photon Flux Density) μMol/M2S is certainly well defined, accepted and consistently used. However, PPF is used inconsistently by nearly every source referencing it."

http://www.inda-gro.com/IG/sites/default/files/pdf/plant-lighting-resource/2-Understanding%20PPF%20and%20PPFD.pdf

"Because the radiation energy intercepted by a surface from a point source is related to the inverse square of the distance between then (Bickford and Dunn, 1972), reducing the distance will have a large impact on the incident light level. Compared with scorching hot, high intensity discharge emitters, cooling LED emitters can be brought much closer to plants tissues. LEDs therefore can be operated at much lower energy levels to give the same incident PPF at the photosynthetic surface."

http://hortsci.ashspublications.org/content/43/7/1951.full

"Lighting terms that do NOT apply to horticulture are below. Some LED manufacturers use these terms and sometimes it can seem like they are more advanced or have something additional to offer, yet when we complete thee research and make a proper educated decision as to our investment; these factors do not need to be considered."

"Lumens, Kelvin Temperature, CRI, CCT, CIE Chromaticity. All these terms are standard lighting measurements that tell us how the light looks to the HUMAN EYE. These terms do not represent the quality of a light spectrum nor do they take into account the McCree Curve."

http://www.eyehortilux.com/education-room/grow-guide.aspx#collapseTwelve

Indeterminate F1 trust tomatoes

"Plants are autotrophs that evolved and use light energy from the sun to create their own food via photosynthesis. Therefore, for LED grow lighting we talk about photosynthetically active radiation (PAR), which is comprised of light between 400-700nanometers in wavelength. We typically measure PAR in photosynthetic photon flux (PPF), measured in **micromoles of photons emitted per second** (micromoles/s). You will also hear us speak of photosynthetic photon flux density (PPFD), which is very useful and measured in **micromoles of photons per square meter per second** (micromoles/s/m^2) to describe the intensity of light particles (i.e., photons) emitted by a LED light at a specific location on a plants canopy."

Zondits Interview with Peter Rumsey, Executive Vive President of Sales and Business Development of LightingScience/VividGro

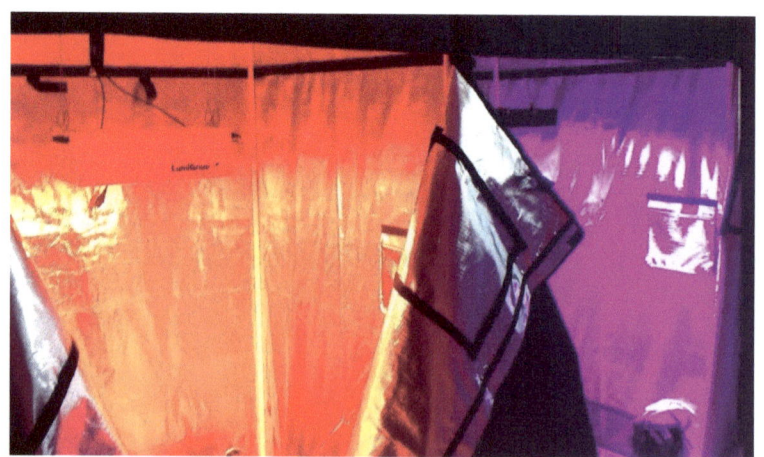

Spectrum Lab

So now let's take a look at some spectrum charts measured from the Lighting Passport from two feet beneath the center of these fixtures, and observe the PPFD measurements at the 450, 660 and 730 nanometer wavelengths. We will start with 450 and move downward respectively. We will also observe a reading from the P3 kill a watt meter to see the energy consumption of each fixture before looking at the PPFD levels. Again, this is so we make proper comparison of a fixtures PPFD output relative to consumption. Is it more difficult to observe the last figure which is 418?

Solar Eclipse 450 AMARE Tech	V2 Lighting Science	Solar System 550 CLW
487	597	418

P3International Kill-A-Watt Meter

450 Nanometer in Wavelength

660 Nanometer in Wavelength

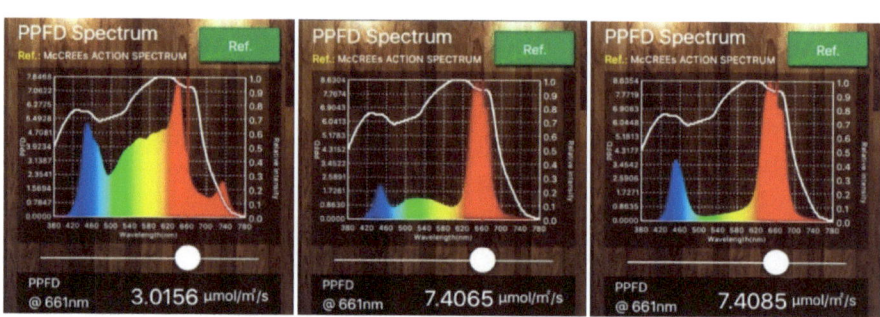

730 Nanometer in Wavelength

Measurements from the Lighting Passport

Parameter	Value	Parameter	Value	Parameter	Value
PPFD (400~700 nm)	1072.5 μmol/m²s	PPFD (400~700 nm)	626.71 μmol/m²s	PPFD (400~700 nm)	672.14 μmol/m²s
PPFD IR (701~780 nm)	81.926 μmol/m²s	PPFD IR (701~780 nm)	14.795 μmol/m²s	PPFD IR (701~780 nm)	17.934 μmol/m²s
PPFD R (600~700 nm)	411.38 μmol/m²s	PPFD R (600~700 nm)	424.06 μmol/m²s	PPFD R (600~700 nm)	483.24 μmol/m²s
PPFD G (500~599 nm)	396.59 μmol/m²s	PPFD G (500~599 nm)	111.40 μmol/m²s	PPFD G (500~599 nm)	46.632 μmol/m²s
PPFD B (400~499 nm)	264.49 μmol/m²s	PPFD B (400~499 nm)	91.273 μmol/m²s	PPFD B (400~499 nm)	142.34 μmol/m²s
PPFD UV (380~399 nm)	1.2161 μmol/m²s	PPFD UV (380~399 nm)	0.5778 μmol/m²s	PPFD UV (380~399 nm)	0.5808 μmol/m²s
YPFD (400~700 nm)	926.49 μmol/m²s	YPFD (400~700 nm)	553.85 μmol/m²s	YPFD (400~700 nm)	592.06 μmol/m²s
YPFD (380~780 nm)	941.69 μmol/m²s	YPFD (380~780 nm)	557.29 μmol/m²s	YPFD (380~780 nm)	596.31 μmol/m²s
YPFD IR (701~780 nm)	14.502 μmol/m²s	YPFD IR (701~780 nm)	3.1062 μmol/m²s	YPFD IR (701~780 nm)	3.9090 μmol/m²s
YPFD R (600~700 nm)	389.98 μmol/m²s	YPFD R (600~700 nm)	393.66 μmol/m²s	YPFD R (600~700 nm)	446.90 μmol/m²s
YPFD G (500~599 nm)	345.59 μmol/m²s	YPFD G (500~599 nm)	93.773 μmol/m²s	YPFD G (500~599 nm)	41.526 μmol/m²s
YPFD B (400~499 nm)	190.92 μmol/m²s	YPFD B (400~499 nm)	66.460 μmol/m²s	YPFD B (400~499 nm)	103.70 μmol/m²s
YPFD UV (380~399 nm)	0.7157 μmol/m²s	YPFD UV (380~399 nm)	0.3393 μmol/m²s	YPFD UV (380~399 nm)	0.3414 μmol/m²s
R/ B	1.56	R/ B	4.65	R/ B	3.39
R/ FR	5.02	R/ FR	28.66	R/ FR	26.95
DLI	92.663 mol/m²	DLI	54.147 mol/m²	DLI	58.073 mol/m²
Illuminance	65461 lux	Illuminance	21696 lux	Illuminance	15573 lux
λp (380~780 nm)	640 nm	λp (380~780 nm)	647 nm	λp (380~780 nm)	647 nm
λD (380~780 nm)	0 nm	λD (380~780 nm)	0 nm	λD (380~780 nm)	0 nm

5. What would you like to see improved on the horticulture LEDs available today? Do you have any advice, recommendations, or suggestions for the LED manufacturers?

"High light output, flexibility in spectrum mixing (so you can produce different recipes), low heat, long lifetimes, flexibility in design and placement are points on which LED designers can work on."

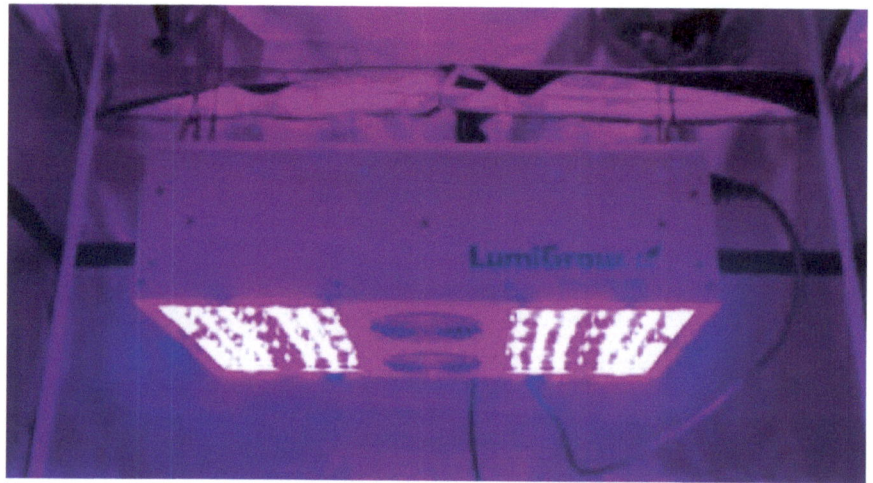

LumiGrow 650 in Spectrum Lab

6. What are some of the pros and cons of using a LED with no cooling fans? Is the energy savings from no fans worth the depreciation of the actual emitters? LEDs with no fans can be just as efficient because the heat syncs are usually heavier and cover more area, hence the heavier fixtures. Also many LEDs that break start having issues with the fan first, once the fan goes the LED diodes quickly overheat and begin diminishing rapidly.

"Passive cooling (without fans) works for 10-20 watts of LEDs in household settings, but running high-power LEDs in close proximity (as needed for growing plants) requires fans to keep the LEDs from degrading."

https://www.blackdogled.com/blog/how-to-compare-different-grow-lights/

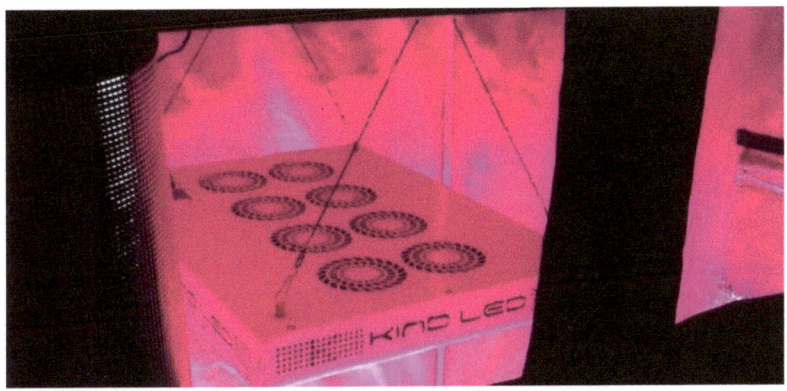

Cooling fans on a K5 1000 KIND LED

7. Some LED manufacturers like Hydrogrow LED, Kind LED, and AMARE Technology are using secondary optics. Others have not used this method. Can you please explain whether or not secondary optics will optimize the light and benefit plants? Or will these secondary optics block light and therefore diminish it? Through the process of transmittance, will the lenses decrease the overall PPFD output? When one considers spectroscopy and optics they begin to see that as light passes through a sample like glass or crystal for example; some light is lost. In the case of a magnification type optic please refer to the figures below.

"It's all related to ppfd variation. If it alters the intended ppfd, then it It's a bad idea, if not then it should not make a difference.

Please refer the below information including measurements or visit the Google Photo album created for the transmittance test of the Solar Eclipse 450 uvb here:

https://goo.gl/photos/457ePZMhMQa58sX96

Strawberry Blond F1

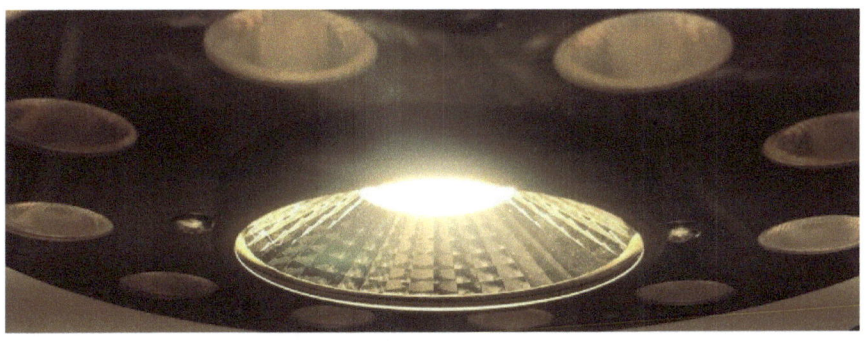

Parameters	Max	Avg	Min
PPFD (400~700 nm)	221.65 μmol/m²s	181.03 μmol/m²s	136.39 μmol/m²s
PPFD IR (701~780 nm)	9.3378 μmol/m²s	7.6587 μmol/m²s	5.9169 μmol/m²s
PPFD R (600~700 nm)	93.646 μmol/m²s	76.580 μmol/m²s	57.855 μmol/m²s
PPFD G (500~599 nm)	97.361 μmol/m²s	79.410 μmol/m²s	59.729 μmol/m²s
PPFD B (400~499 nm)	30.634 μmol/m²s	25.034 μmol/m²s	18.803 μmol/m²s
PPFD UV (380~399 nm)	0.1742 μmol/m²s	0.1486 μmol/m²s	0.1024 μmol/m²s
YPFD (400~700 nm)	97.427 μmol/m²s	79.622 μmol/m²s	59.968 μmol/m²s
YPFD (380~780 nm)	97.501 μmol/m²s	79.683 μmol/m²s	60.011 μmol/m²s
YPFD IR (701~780 nm)	0.0000 μmol/m²s	0.0000 μmol/m²s	0.0000 μmol/m²s
YPFD R (600~700 nm)	45.615 μmol/m²s	37.319 μmol/m²s	28.177 μmol/m²s
YPFD G (500~599 nm)	28.454 μmol/m²s	23.210 μmol/m²s	17.456 μmol/m²s
YPFD B (400~499 nm)	23.347 μmol/m²s	19.083 μmol/m²s	14.327 μmol/m²s
YPFD UV (380~399 nm)	0.0728 μmol/m²s	0.0603 μmol/m²s	0.0416 μmol/m²s
R/B	3.09	3.06	3.04
R/IR	10.23	9.98	9.78
DLI	19.151 mol/m²	15.641 mol/m²	11.784 mol/m²
Illuminance	15406 lux	12569 lux	9459 lux
λp (380~780 nm)	601 nm	600 nm	600 nm
λD (380~780 nm)	581 nm	581 nm	581 nm
CCT	3466 K	3457 K	3447 K
CRI (Ra)	84	84	84

Parameters	Max	Avg	Min
PPFD (400~700 nm)	385.49 µmol/m²s	313.73 µmol/m²s	184.67 µmol/m²s
PPFD IR (701~780 nm)	16.248 µmol/m²s	13.331 µmol/m²s	8.1125 µmol/m²s
PPFD R (600~700 nm)	162.88 µmol/m²s	132.83 µmol/m²s	79.169 µmol/m²s
PPFD G (500~599 nm)	169.37 µmol/m²s	137.91 µmol/m²s	81.254 µmol/m²s
PPFD B (400~499 nm)	53.227 µmol/m²s	42.975 µmol/m²s	24.234 µmol/m²s
PPFD UV (380~399 nm)	0.3245 µmol/m²s	0.2609 µmol/m²s	0.1327 µmol/m²s
YPFD (400~700 nm)	169.41 µmol/m²s	137.77 µmol/m²s	80.722 µmol/m²s
YPFD (380~780 nm)	169.53 µmol/m²s	137.88 µmol/m²s	80.777 µmol/m²s
YPFD IR (701~780 nm)	0.0000 µmol/m²s	0.0000 µmol/m²s	0.0000 µmol/m²s
YPFD R (600~700 nm)	79.337 µmol/m²s	64.708 µmol/m²s	38.562 µmol/m²s
YPFD G (500~599 nm)	49.492 µmol/m²s	40.307 µmol/m²s	23.757 µmol/m²s
YPFD B (400~499 nm)	40.563 µmol/m²s	32.743 µmol/m²s	18.394 µmol/m²s
YPFD UV (380~399 nm)	0.1320 µmol/m²s	0.1052 µmol/m²s	0.0533 µmol/m²s
R/B	3.27	3.11	3.02
R/IR	10.11	9.95	9.76
DLI	33.306 mol/m²	27.106 mol/m²	15.955 mol/m²
Illuminance	26795 lux	21820 lux	12869 lux
λp (380~780 nm)	601 nm	600 nm	600 nm
λD (380~780 nm)	581 nm	581 nm	581 nm
CCT	3472 K	3445 K	3399 K
CRI (Ra)	84	84	84

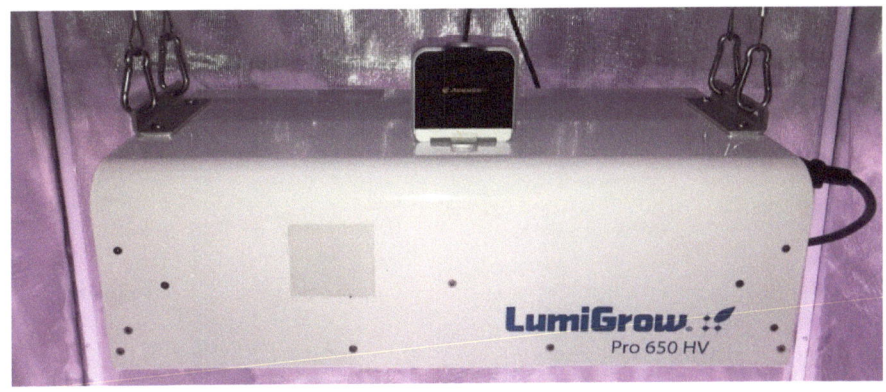

Parameters	Max	Avg	Min
PPFD (400~700 nm)	343.98 μmol/m²s	331.71 μmol/m²s	304.11 μmol/m²s
PPFD IR (701~780 nm)	8.9947 μmol/m²s	8.4113 μmol/m²s	7.3780 μmol/m²s
PPFD R (600~700 nm)	265.69 μmol/m²s	255.24 μmol/m²s	232.95 μmol/m²s
PPFD G (500~599 nm)	15.474 μmol/m²s	14.960 μmol/m²s	13.797 μmol/m²s
PPFD B (400~499 nm)	63.014 μmol/m²s	61.538 μmol/m²s	57.398 μmol/m²s
PPFD UV (380~399 nm)	0.3494 μmol/m²s	0.3101 μmol/m²s	0.2302 μmol/m²s
YPFD (400~700 nm)	303.45 μmol/m²s	292.70 μmol/m²s	268.39 μmol/m²s
YPFD (380~780 nm)	305.52 μmol/m²s	294.72 μmol/m²s	270.16 μmol/m²s
YPFD IR (701~780 nm)	1.9372 μmol/m²s	1.8338 μmol/m²s	1.6167 μmol/m²s
YPFD R (600~700 nm)	243.03 μmol/m²s	233.70 μmol/m²s	213.51 μmol/m²s
YPFD G (500~599 nm)	13.819 μmol/m²s	13.363 μmol/m²s	12.319 μmol/m²s
YPFD B (400~499 nm)	46.764 μmol/m²s	45.665 μmol/m²s	42.593 μmol/m²s
YPFD UV (380~399 nm)	0.2055 μmol/m²s	0.1822 μmol/m²s	0.1369 μmol/m²s
R/B	4.22	4.15	4.01
R/IR	31.64	30.38	28.65
DLI	29.720 mol/m²	28.660 mol/m²	26.275 mol/m²
Illuminance	5312 lux	5132 lux	4704 lux
λp (380~780 nm)	664 nm	662 nm	661 nm
λD (380~780 nm)	0 nm	0 nm	0 nm
CCT	7321 K	6908 K	6055 K
CRI (Ra)	-73	-78	-80

LumiGrow 650 Ten point measurement comparison

"Transmittance is the fraction of incident light at a specified wavelength that passes through a sample. Transmittance is measured in percent and is used to specify the light throughput of transparent material. Transmittance Rate- is the physical process of light passing through a sample."

"Allied Scientific Pro from both offices in Canada and Taiwan (R.O.C.) have 13 years of expertise in optical components and assemblies in the photonics market. We have qualified over the years a few key optics suppliers in Canada, USA and lately Taiwan and China for the best of the quality and price solutions."

https://alliedscientificpro.com/shop/product/custom-optical-components-and-assembly-19247

Another thought would be using a system to automatically lower and raise grow lights as the project manager sees fit. This can add additional savings to the HVAC expenses while increasing the quality and quantity of the harvest.

"The motorized Sun winch allows you to raise and lower your light fixtures from up to 30 feet away using a wireless remote! Make quick and easy adjustments to the position of your light fixtures with this motorized lift system for your lighting fixtures."

https://4hydroponics.com/sun-winch-motorized-lift

https://youtu.be/KaWTaEeBCy4

https://www.google.com/patents/US20150351325

Optics on the V1 from Lighting Science

"Secondary lenses focus the light to give it an impressive PAR, YPF or other intensity measurement, but only at a single point, destroying the light's total growing footprint and losing about 10% of the light in the process."

"Secondary lenses for LEDs are designed to refocus the light from the diode and primary lens into a new, usually narrower beam. Many LED grow light companies are using secondary lenses and claim to "amplify", "magnify", or "boost the output of" the light. The secondary lenses are magnifying the light in exactly the same way a magnifying glass does in the sun- but no additional light is being produced or "harvested" from the LED, it is just being focused to a narrower beam or even a point. In fact, about 10% of the light is reflected or refracted by the secondary lens and is lost- but the remaining 90% gets focused into a more-intense beam."

https://www.blackdogled.com/blog/how-to-compare-different-grow-lights/

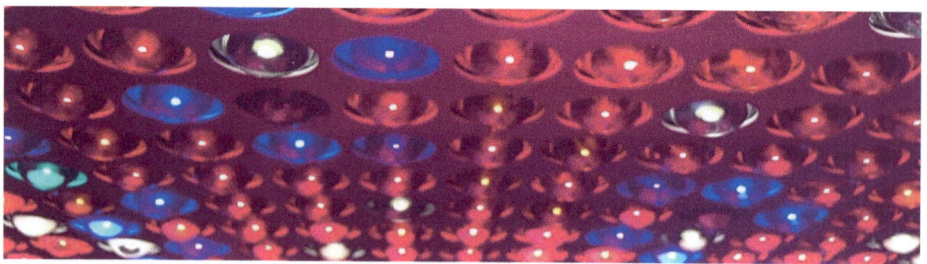

Secondary Optics

8. When we consider the two primary areas of the spectrum that influence photosynthesis; Is it safe to say that these white light LEDs are not as effective as the Red Blue spectrum LEDs?

There is still a use and space in the market for white light LEDs. Some growers prefer to use MH bulbs throughout the vegetative and flowering cycles of their project, and these white light LEDs are a common choice for these MH growers. Now some of the horticulturists that enjoy experimenting with different spectra will often find the Red/Blue LEDs with adjustment capability more desirable. Either way it's still essential for us to recall the two primary areas of photosynthetic response when it comes to spectra.

"Plants under 660nm and 470nm LEDs sustained higher leaf photosynthetic rates."

http://hortsci.ashspublications.org/content/43/7/1951.full

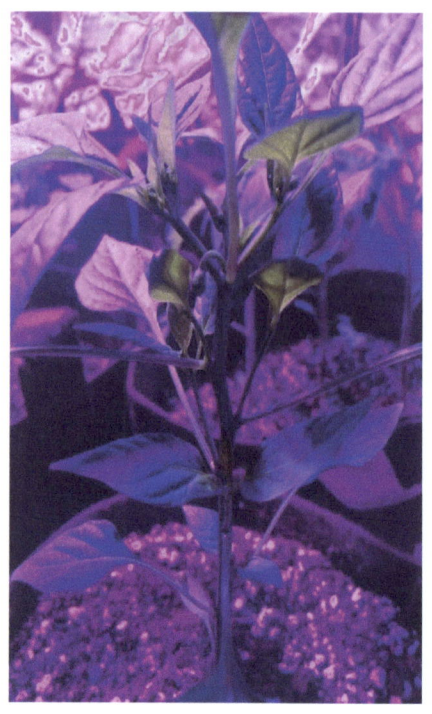

"Broadband sources, including the sun, also emit more than what is required for photosynthesis. Much of this light results in heat, which is crippling to a plants performance if the temperature of the environment is elevated what plants can tolerate. With LEDs users can now pick out specific red and blue wavelengths ideal for photosynthesis, thereby eliminating the excess light that produces excess heat."

The experiment from the Max Yield article focused on the wavelengths associated with photosynthesis 425-470nm-625-650nm. Please keep in mind this article was published in 2010.

Max Yield July 2010 by Brian Chiang and Josh Pucket

F1 Trust & Strawberry Blond floral development

"Plants preferentially absorb red and blue light. Much of the light produced by "white" LEDs are in spectra (colors) that plants do not use. This unused light is just converted to heat within the leaves, requiring lower environmental temperatures to maintain optimal leaf surface temperatures. When combined with the 20%-40% efficiency loss, white LEDs are less than half as efficient for growing plants than the correct mix of pure-color LEDs-- white LED grow lights force you to cool your growing environment more, just like HPS and MH, losing a lot of the other advantages LEDs offer."

"Almost all "white" LEDs on the market today are actually just a blue LED with a phosphor coating which converts much of the blue light into different colors. The most commonly available "white" LEDs use a phosphor called Yttrium Aluminium Garnet (YAG) which predominantly creates yellow light; the combination looks white to the human eye and has a much better Color Rendition Index (CRI) than RGB LEDs due to the wider spectrum created by the phosphor. However, 20%-40% of the light produced by the blue LED is lost in this process, so these "white" LEDs cannot be as efficient at creating light as a pure-color LED."

https://www.blackdogled.com/blog/led-types/

"The advantages to quality grow LEDs far outweigh the drawbacks now, including the following; 40% + energy consumption (kWh) reduction, greatly reduced waste heat output (reducing HVAC loads), low to no maintenance, available rebates, optimized spectrum and intensity for increased crop quality, reduced grow cycle time, and increased crop yields. Note that the reduced heat output of LED fixtures means that they can be positioned closer to the canopy and provide higher PAR levels without cooking the plant"

Zondits Interview with Peter Rumsey, Executive Vive President of Sales and Business Development of LightingScience/VividGro

F1 Tomato cluster grown with a Solar System 550

9. Which wattage LED emitters 1,3, or 5 watt are most efficient for which sort of application?

"Many LED grow light resellers have entered the market and in an effort to differentiate themselves some have turned to the 5 watt and 10 watt diode chips. These larger diodes have shortcomings when it comes to indoor growing. The larger chips give off more heat and require more heat dissipation. They need larger heat sinks and make for a heavier product. The 5 watt and 10 watt diodes also require the grow light to be larger because they cannot be manufactured in a dense network like the 3 watt diode chips."

http://www.dormgrow.com/blog/

" 5W diodes are brighter still and provide canopy-penetration equivalent to or better than a 1000W HID light."

https://www.blackdogled.com/blog/led-types/

Kind LED Secondary Optics

10. What is the optimum PPFD for a plant outside? As we move toward indoor PFALs and begin supplementing the air with CO2; what is the ideal PPFD for the different levels of CO2?

"Being able to move the light source closer to the plants means we can reach higher PAR levels than HID lighting. This, in turn means that our customers can push the metabolism and growth rate of the plants very close to their genetic maximum. Also we must take extra care to mind the other limiting variables to photosynthesis to include temperature, humidity, media moisture, CO2 levels, and especially nutrient levels."

Zondits Interview with Peter Rumsey, Executive Vive President of Sales and Business Development of LightingScience/VividGro

http://onlinelibrary.wiley.com/doi/10.1111/j.1751-1097.1987.tb04757.x/abstract

https://www.ncbi.nlm.nih.gov/pmc/articles/PMC3550641/pdf/12298_2008_Article_27.pdf

"Photosynthesis occurs inside of specialized organelles known as chloroplasts, and is the process that uses light energy to split water (H_2O) and fix carbon dioxide (CO_2) to produce carbohydrates (CH_2O) and oxygen (O_2). The process is very complex; however, a simple diagram of the reaction is shown in Figure 3. As light intensity (PPFD) increases, photosynthetic rates also increase until a saturation point is reached. Every plant species has a light saturation point where photosynthetic levels plateau. Light saturation normally occurs when some other factor (normally CO_2) is limited"

TABLE 3: RECOMMENDED PPFD ($\mu mol/m^2/s$)

Species	Establishment		Vegetative	Reproductive
	Seed	Vegetative Cutting		
Cannabis	100-300	75-150	300-600	600+
Tomatoes	150-350	75-150	350-600	600+
Cucumbers	100-300	--	300-600	600+
Peppers	150-350	--	300-600	600+

Fluence Bioengineering_High PPFD Cultivation Guide_v1.2 (1)

"Carbon dioxide (CO2) enrichment in your controlled environment will substantially improve the yield of your high PPFD crops. All plants have a light saturation point where the maximum rate of photosynthesis is reached at a specific light intensity. Maximum photosynthesis at ambient atmospheric CO2 levels (~400 ppm) is normally limited by the amount of CO2 available, not the intensity of light (Figure 5). Generally, optimum levels of CO2 will be two to four times the normal atmospheric levels (800 – 1,400 ppm CO2) when growing under high PPFD conditions. We recommend supplementing ≥ 800 ppm CO2 into your controlled environment when you are providing your plants with ≥ 500 μmol/m2/s. As you increase your light intensity, you can slowly increase your CO2 levels as plants acclimate to increased PPFD. Refer to Table 4 for recommended CO2 concentrations during establishment, vegetative, and reproductive growth of cannabis, tomatoes, cucumbers, and peppers."

LED Floral Development

Species	Establishment	Vegetative	Reproductive
Cannabis	400	400-800	800-1400
Tomatoes	400	400-800	700-1200
Cucumbers	400-600	400-800	800-1000
Peppers	400-600	400-800	800-1000

Figure 5: Influence of CO_2 concentration on the rate of photosynthesis.

Fluence Bioengineering_High PPFD Cultivation Guide_v1.2 (1)

Is there a benefit to having consistent UV in the spectrum throughout the plants entire life cycle? UVA or UVB…

"High concentrations of ultraviolet light have been associated with induction of anthocyanin (Krizek et al., 1998). The addition of the blue light significantly increased the concentration of anthocanin in the leaf tissue as well as altered the developmental morphology."

http://hortsci.ashspublications.org/content/44/2/231.full

Are there better, more precise UV applications in floriculture; like using UV for last two weeks of a flower cycle, or an EOD (end of day) treatment?

Ultra Violet or UV is measured in illuminance or (Lux) and Spectral Irradiance (mW/m^2) which is different from the commonly seen PPF, PPFD, and DLI abbreviations. Keep in mind traditional lighting measurements such as Lumens, PAR and Kelvin temperature do not measure UV. Only a UV meter or a spectral distribution chart can provide the correct information on a light source's UV output. UV light is divided up into three sections. UVA=400nm-315nm, UVB=315nm-280nm, UVC=280nm-100nm.

UVB light is the most significant cause factor for cancer. UVB light will not penetrate human skin like the UVA can, and doesn't have the same reaction response as UVC, but still UVB is the major cause of cancer around the world. So, before we go rushing out to purchase UVB supplementary lighting for our horticulture projects let's make sure we understand it, what it can do, and how we can safely use in to be a beneficial contribute to the garden.

UVB light has been proven to stimulate protomorphic effects that change a plants biochemical composition. UVB light has been shown to effect the photosynthetic competence, stimulate defensive mechanisms, and change the morphogenesis of certain species. There is also UVR8 which is a protein in the plant that senses UVB light specifically influencing cryptochrome and the other flavonoids. UVR8 is a photoreceptor and can signal certain responses through signaling pathways. UVB photons are high energy and can overpower and burn the photosynthetic apparatus and cell walls of the plant. It's always advised to exercise restraint from using UV radiation until one has some experience with the applications.

Cryptochrome are a specific family of flavoproteins that are sensitive to blue light. They are found in plants and animals. Cryptochromes are involved in the circadian rhythms of plants and animals, and possibly also in the sensing of magnetic fields in a number of species. Cryptochrome is a very important aspect to consider especially when contemplating using UVB light in your operation.

UV light will stress most plants cell surface and can actually burn the cell wall and the photosynthesis apparatus; it can burn the leaves and cause all kinds of harm to the cell walls. UVB stress in moderation has a mild negative effect, but them stimulates the plant to come back and repair and damage and increase its defensive mechanism. Trichomes are one of the defensive mechanisms of the Cannabis Sativa which provides multiple medicinal opportunities, so the study of UV application in horticulture has enormous potential.

In certain fruits and vegetables the presence of mild UVB initially stresses the leaf surface, and then again stimulates a repair and defensive response. Some horticulturists have found that this response can be pigment stimulation or color change. There can also be increased antioxidant properties in the fruit, and the plant can also accumulate larger amounts of DNA repair enzymes. There are many different things that UV light can do to your plants.

There is growing popularity when it comes to UVB for horticultural lighting purposes, especially for Cannabis. This has different application rates from research to researcher, although it seems everyone is on the same page when it comes to using UVB during the final two weeks of flowering. UVB can increase photosynthesis and can actually cause burning or damage to the photosynthetic apparatus and stomata. To be same we can measure the sunlight and see the luminance levels of UVB outside and them we can try to mimic this inside our greenhouses or labs. It's always best to be cautious when increasing UVB levels above what we normally observe outdoors. There are many different applications for UVB that vary between crops and plant lifecycle.

UVB has also been shown to increase pigmentation and color in flowers. Pigments are wavelength specific so this will be a finding that many researchers will continue looking at in the future. UVB is also used for vegetative growth especially in species like Cannabis Sativa like Arjan's strawberry haze and Arjan's haze #3. UVB can also be used in the spectrum for growing indeterminate tomatoes like F1 Trust. UVB helps drive photosynthesis, shortening, and tight intermodal spacing by stimulating and influencing cryptochrome. One thing it seems everyone can agree on is the fact that UVB radiation triggers the production and extensive development of THC in those varieties specifically bead for high THC content. And it's this factor alone that is driving the increasing desire for gardeners to implement UVB light into their gardens.

A general way to think about UV stress having a positive effect on your plants is the outdoor transplant situation where your crops are scheduled to go outside yet still need some hardening off before taking on the full sun. Applying some UVB during the week leading up to the transplant outside will help the plant prepare for what's going to happen in the future.

Unfortunately there are some risk factors that need to be considered before adding a UVB light to the system.

Some of the main questions cultivators experimenting with UV stress find themselves asking are; is there a benefit to having consistent UV in the spectrum throughout the plants entire life cycle? Are there better, more precise UV applications in floriculture; using UV in vegetative to keep plants compact, using UV stress to harden off before transplanting, using UV stress for last two weeks of a flower cycle, or a BOD treatment?

According to Ashs Publications on UVB Increasing the illuminance of UVB onto the canopy can influence the induction of anthocyanin, also the addition of the blue light significantly increased the concentration of anthocanin in the leaf tissue as well as changed the plants overall rate of photosynthesis, developmental, and morphology.

UV light stresses the plants, yet it's this stress from UVA and UVB that plays a vital role in many aspects of plant growth. Plants in nature will be exposed to sunlight which includes high levels of UVA and UVB. Many of the artificial lighting sources today used for indoor plant growth produce very small amounts of UV or don't produce any at all.

Natural sunlight produces these three sections of UV. However, UVC is not naturally present on earth because the Earth's atmosphere blocks the extremely harmful light from reaching the Earth's surface. One of the most popular research articles on UV light is the previously released study on Cannabis Sativa which was printed in Great Britain. UV-B radiation effects on photosynthesis, growth and cannabinoid production of two Cannabis Sativa chemotypes; has been one of the foundational papers on the using UV light for medicinal application.

Lighting sources can artificially produce all three types of UV; however the components used to construct the light source, such as glass, will generally block UV emitted from the light. This is essential for greenhouse growers to understand as the lack of UV inside greenhouses due to the glass has been contributed to the lack of taste and nutrition in greenhouse tomatoes. Check the spectral distribution chart on your grow lamps packaging to see if your light is producing any UV.

UV light stresses the plants and this reaction to the UV stress activates the plant's defense mechanisms. Creating increased amounts of terpenes and tricomes are only two effects UV stress can have on plants. UV causes plants to produce oils, antioxidant vitamins and flavonoids to protect themselves from the damaging effects of UV like its natural sunblock. Greenhouses block the UV portion of the spectrum from entering, and many tomato farmers and taste testers have found that using supplemental UV light will increase flavor in the out of season greenhouse varieties. UV seems to increase smell, flavor, and taste in many different plant types. UVB also stimulates the anthocyanins which are the blue, violet, or red flavonoid pigment found in plants.

These compounds produce the vibrant colors, smells and tastes of your plants. If your light source does not produce UV, you are effectively changing the color, smell and taste of your crop. Knowing how to safely and effectively apply UV light to your garden will keep power and control in your hands and greatly increase the attractiveness of your harvest.

UVB light will stress your plants; it's this UVB stress that has the ability to stimulate certain secondary plant metabolites such as flavonoids, poluphenolic compounds, terpenes, and cannaboids. This is done by stimulating the cryptochrome pathways that are responsible for initiating the production of the metabolites. Also UVB light will contribute to the characteristics one might see from using a heavy blue spectrum. The plants will be short, compact, and bushy. UVB and Blue 450nm both contribute to these characteristics and UVB and Blue also have a synergetic effect when used together making the two a powerful tool for cultivators working with long varieties that like to stretch out. Now from using Blue 450nm and UVB these varieties can be grown in denser more compact forms, creating a more efficient use of production space.

UVB is used today by advanced cultivators to increase trichomes and terpene profiles; which would be any of a large group of volatile unsaturated hydrocarbons found in the essential oils of plants, especially conifers and citrus trees. They are based on a cyclic molecule having the formula C_{10H16}

For some growers Terpenes is a new term that's being thrown around in the industry quite frequently these days. Terpenes are a diverse class of organic compounds produced by a variety of plants, and some insects. Many terpenes are aromatic and may create a form of protection for the plant and are the major building blocks of Resin and essential oils. Terpenes and "terpenoids" are the primary components of the essential oils that are being harvested for the medicinal properties like CBD, there are many different types of terpenes that come from a variety of plants and flowers.

Plants will naturally product and use terpenes for a range of functions from temperature regulation, metabolism, respiration, and pest control. A range of terpenes have even been identified as high-value chemicals in food, cosmetic, pharmaceutical and biotechnology industries, the only issue is that plants produce such a small percentage of terpenes, making them difficult time consuming and expensive to extract them. Some UVB lighting sill help growers increase their terpene profiles and extraction levels.

The average high terpene levels run at about 2%. Most recently though, there have been many studies done around Terpenes and a particular company using achieved a terpene level of 3.78! Many different lighting companies are focusing their research and development assets on UV and how it can be safely incorporated into the project. Solis-Tek also has an additive product called Terpenez which is specifically used for increasing the terpene profile in medicional varieties. Over 100 commercial growers have done controlled and non-controlled side-by-side testing with Terpenez and have seen significant results. Terpenez is made from all organic and natural compounds and contains no heavy metals.

UV stress being used at the end of the plants lifecycle contributes to the overall terpene profile. Not only do terpenes contribute significantly to smell, texture, and flavor; but they also can be used for everything from a natural pesticide, fungal deterrent, and warning sign to intruding animals.

UV light is the most dangerous for human eyes; it can affect the cons and rods in the eye which may distort color and depth perception. Also UV is known to contribute to cataracts and macular degeneration; which is why we always recommend using the proper eye protection equipment from Method Seven.

One last note on UV is that all plants have evolved over the centuries with the presence of UV which means that many different plant species have found different ways to protect themselves from it. UV applications have been found to increase terpenes, general medicinal properties like CBD, and UV has been found to help tomato plants avoid disease in greenhouses.

As we move from UV applications and start looking at full spectrums please keep in mind that plants number one driving force is the light. Plants contain many different types of photoreceptors that sense and utilize light. These include crytochromes, phytochromes, and phototrophins. Each react to different wavelengths and the ratio of their active and inactive forms cause different reactions in plants Many people believe that the nutrients are what has the most significant effect on the plant which is actually incorrect, it the light. The light contributes significantly to driving photosynthesis and thus growth rate, and also signals messages to the plant like what season or time of day it is. Lighting also influences the plants metabolism and helps the plant consume carbon dioxide; the amount of light determines how much water will be required that day and what PH it should be at. Light and photoperiod also drive the plant to uptake certain nutrients. For example, some growers use T5 cool white florescent for early vegetative phase and they keep the lights on from 16-24 hours a day depending on the gardener's preferences. This T5 light spectrum and photoperiod drive vegetative growth and signal that the plant needs high levels on Nitrogen. The 12/12 photoperiod with a HPS spectrum will signal a very different nutrient requirement to your plants, they will need increased PPM levels of Phosphorous and Potassium. Understanding light and the different photoperiods can create new opportunities for cultivators at every level.

Overexposure is certainly a risk factor that must be considered. When considering the use of UV light; what amounts and which types of plants are best suited for the environment are two critical questions. Its beneficial to look at where that specific variety of plant derived from because knowing its place of origin can help determine its natural UV levels from the sun. Reviewing a global chart of the hemispheres and understanding the change of seasons relative to El Niño is also very helpful. Then we can have a much better idea of what that type can handle. One can also measure the sunlight outside with a UV Illuminance Spectrometer, or read over this book and find what UV levels are appropriate for their design.

Questions answered in part by **Dr. Rez Mani** application scientist of York University Canada

Detailed answers in red are from Dr. Mani:

http://www.yorku.ca/index.html

Zondits Interview with **Peter Rumsey**, Executive Vive President of Sales and Business Development of LightingScience/VividGro

Answers in blue are from Peter Rumsey of Lighting Science

https://www.lsgc.com/

https://vividgro.com/

Answers in green from Blackdog LED

https://www.blackdogled.com/blog/led-types/

https://www.ncbi.nlm.nih.gov/pmc/articles/PMC3550641/pdf/12298_2008_Article_27.pdf

Max Yield July 2010 by Brian Chiang and Josh Pucket

http://hortsci.ashspublications.org/content/43/7/1951.full

https://oup.silverchair-cdn.com/oup/backfile/Content_public/Journal/pcp/50/4/10.1093/pcp/pcp034/2/pcp034.pdf?Expires=1493256339&Signature=V5DVH6t5d7nSO5feZ~Zfv0X78Audop7MZLsVjibqCqDzMXUg9hmcPUXD9tdlUKV7TNLJh-TlYDpGSVqKbyt3kj0g4uIoErfidLbVCe9xriD5OcSiUsjHvRB6uFTtRsi1Ef2fZgC51ZP2BNO~DFTE1KVdQl8teBuHre~TDvs1iFrBM3bSq9AQgmhoauJ7hI0IzoH6GoUUcLrKjYfq57stKEEJcbcboGermjadPiNO4~BMWoM8DxgcqJ-I0II32rpqYzOgt9rY2f9b2jXyfCpXPaRwv9c0HKaYnypW-YtrlVMt-7SzZMB1q3qnkkIId~9qDHDHtM9Lhh4YfUhHpqTJ-g__&Key-Pair-Id=APKAIUCZBIA4LVPAVW3Q

http://onlinelibrary.wiley.com/doi/10.1111/j.1751-1097.1987.tb04757.x/abstract

https://4hydroponics.com/sun-winch-motorized-lift

https://youtu.be/KaWTaEeBCy4

https://www.google.com/patents/US20150351325

https://alliedscientificpro.com/shop/product/custom-optical-components-and-assembly-19247

http://www.dormgrow.com/blog/

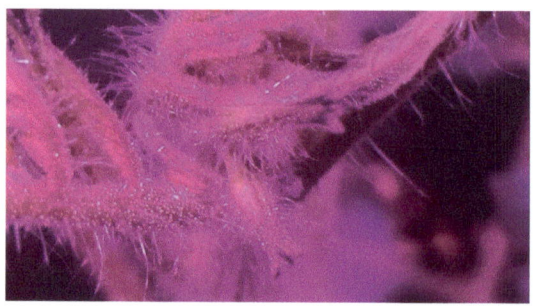

F1 Trust Tomato flower development under the G8-900

Additional Resources include;

http://www.hortimax.com/7/18/89/en/news/hortimax-launches-new-uv-disinfection-unit.html

http://www.hortimax.nl/7/18/88/en/news/help!-were-running-out-of-phosphorus.html

http://www.ledhorticulture.com/hello-world/

http://www.ledhorticulture.com/why-is-led-lighting-so-good-for-plants/

http://www.ledhorticulture.com/the-significance-of-light-quality-in-cultivation/

https://alliedscientificpro.com/blog/our-news-1/post/photometrics-level-1-webinar-_32#blog_content

Four readings recommended by Dr. Mani:

https://www.researchgate.net/publication/10938361_Improving_spinach_radish_and_lettuce_growth_under_red_LEDs_with_blue_light_supplementation?enrichId=rgreq-596baf40-8189-454b-a084-56fbfe52c637&enrichSource=Y292ZXJQYWdlOzEwOTM4MzYxO0FTOjE5ODU2NDg1MzYyMDczNkAxNDI0MzUyOTU4MzY4&el=1_x_2

https://www.researchgate.net/publication/7963634_Green-light_Supplementation_for_Enhanced_Lettuce_Growth_under_Red-_and_Blue-light-emitting_Diodes?enrichId=rgreq-13a41f01-a70b-4445-9b30-c21e575245d9&enrichSource=Y292ZXJQYWdlOzc5NjM2MzQ7QVM6MTk4NTY0ODUzNjIwNzM4QDE0MjQzNTI5NTkwMDc%3D&el=1_x_2

Applications of Far-Red LEDs in Plant Production under Controlled Enviroments **Chieri Kubota**

http://hortsci.ashspublications.org/content/44/2/231.full

www.ingramcontent.com/pod-product-compliance
Lightning Source LLC
Chambersburg PA
CBHW040235220526
45473CB00001B/254